SKIN CARE
FOR PSORIASIS

The author and publishers welcome feedback from the users of this book. Please contact the publishers:

Class Publishing,
Barb House, Barb Mews,
London W6 7PA, UK
Telephone: 0171 371 2119
Fax: 0171 371 2878 [International +44171]

Printing history:
Class Publishing:
First edition 1997

A CIP catalogue record for this book is available from the British Library

ISBN 1 872362 63 X

Edited by Ruth Midgley
Designed by Wendy Bann
Typesetting by Louise Dick, Ruth Midgley
Production by Landmark Production Consultants Ltd,
  Princes Risborough
Printed and bound in Great Britain by Clays Ltd, St Ives plc

SKIN CARE
FOR PSORIASIS

Dr. V.K. Dave, FRCP

Honorary Consultant Dermatologist
Dermatology Centre
Hope Hospital, Salford

CLASS PUBLISHING • LONDON

ACKNOWLEDGEMENTS

Thanks are due to all the nursing staff at the Dermatology Centre, Hope Hospital, Salford for their detailed contributions to the skin care routines described. The preparation of the manuscript by Mrs Susan Parkinson and the editorial assistance of Ms Ruth Midgley are gratefully acknowledged.

SKIN RESEARCH CENTRE
University of Manchester

Many skin problems have yet to be examined by advanced research techniques. This Centre provides a forum for research into conditions ranging from eczema and psoriasis to skin cancer and wound healing. It is jointly organised by the medical and the scientific staff in the University.

The sale of this book supports research into skin conditions.

FOREWORD

by Christopher E. M. Griffiths, B.Sc, MD, FRCP, Professor of Dermatology, University of Manchester

Psoriasis takes its name from the Greek word "psora", meaning "the itch". It is a common condition, known to affect 2 to 3% of the UK population. In fact, the true percentage may be higher – it has been calculated that only 20% of sufferers actually consult a doctor about it.

Despite a considerable amount of research, a cure for psoriasis still seems only a distant promise. Current treatments do no more than suppress the condition. Consequently, the way individuals cope with their condition is of paramount importance.

At present, very few publications address what people with psoriasis can do for themselves to complement the medicines and other treatments prescribed by their doctors. Dr V.K. Dave has many years' experience as a consultant dermatologist and has a particular interest in psoriasis. His self-help book provides practical tips to help alleviate the day-to-day suffering and inconvenience of psoriasis. Much of the personal advice included in this book has already appeared in patient leaflets used in Dr Dave's practice over many years. Practical advice based on experience is often what works best.

I am sure that anyone who has psoriasis, or who has family members with psoriasis, will benefit from reading this easy-to-follow and practical self-help guide.

INTRODUCTION

When psoriasis appears in the skin, it causes intense frustration, especially to the young.

This book is written for the many whose psoriasis is mild or in its early stages. The psychological effects of psoriasis are particularly disturbing at its onset. The distress makes the problem worse. A vicious circle, in which psoriasis and stress interact, can easily develop. Detailed guidance on self care routines, particularly when psoriasis is at an early stage, often makes it possible to control the rash. This belief is the reason for writing this book.

The importance of self care in the treatment of psoriasis is not a new concept. Long before effective drugs became available, the medical profession relied almost exclusively on an holistic approach to control psoriasis. The individual's lifestyle was carefully assessed, and suitable advice given, before any drug treatment was organised. Such guidance may, however, be of little benefit to the small group of people whose psoriasis requires close medical supervision.

Psoriasis can be a major cosmetic problem, especially to women. This book, therefore, includes a great deal of practical advice on skin care. The routines described are well known to the nursing staff in hospital skin clinics. Such information has been collected here so that it can be made more widely available. The book also compensates for the fact that it is often impractical to discuss many of its points during medical consultations.

Very few medical facts about psoriasis are discussed in this book. Complex scientific ideas are deliberately set out simply and directly. Medical terms, too, have been largely avoided. The instructions relate only to the common patterns of psoriasis. No allowance has been made for exceptions. Some of the advice included reflects personal observations. It is hoped that this book will signpost the road to control over psoriasis.

HOW TO USE THIS BOOK

This book doesn't discuss all the facts about psoriasis, or offer guidance to everyone with this condition, or describe its medical treatment, or claim to give any new answers to the problem.

What this book does is tell you what you can do to make your skin more comfortable, and how you can take control of the problem so that psoriasis doesn't rule your life.

Aim to read the whole book. The advice is written in a concentrated form, so it may be best to read a few chapters at a time. Then follow the instructions in the chapters that apply to you.

The early sections mostly offer general advice. Detailed information follows on. Where useful, basic simple advice is repeated. The aim is to fix the important points in your mind. You can then work out solutions that suit your own needs.

CONTENTS

1 SELF-HELP AND PSORIASIS

Psoriasis can be a nuisance in many ways. However, there is a great deal you can do to control the condition. The self-help measures described in this book have two basic aims:

1 To help your skin heal quickly.

2 To help it remain healed for a long time.

You will find that much of the advice given is based on common-sense. This should help you to remember it – and also to achieve the best results.

Variations in the Rash

Psoriasis shows up differently in different people. In most people, the rash appears in only a few areas of the body. This is not likely to change. Don't imagine that your rash will spread to all the areas of the body described in this book. For example, very few people develop psoriasis on their hands, feet and face or in their joints.

The Importance of Self-help

In someone with psoriasis, the skin has certain characteristic features:

1   It doesn't tolerate damage from stretching.

2   Its ability to retain moisture is altered.

3   It becomes inflamed when there is infection in the body folds.

4   Its immune reactions are modified.

Self-help measures can affect how successfully your skin counters these changes. This is the basic theme of the book.

Self-help and Medical Treatment

Self-help measures for people with psoriasis are described at length in the chapters that follow. Much of the advice relates to practical skin care, but other aspects – such as lifestyle and the possible role of allergies – are also considered.

The guide-lines given in this book should add to the instructions you receive from your doctor or at your local clinic. Although there are common patterns in psoriasis, there are also many variations. The medical treatment you receive needs to suit your skin and also to be appropriate for your particular type of psoriasis.

The self-help advice in this book has been carefully written so that following it will not make your problem worse. If you are at all uncertain on this, discuss the instructions with your medical adviser (see also Appendix 4). It is also possible that you don't have to follow all the advice offered in this book. The treatment prescribed for the rash may clear it and the problem may disappear.

Lifestyle, Allergies and Yeasts

Any of these factors can complicate psoriasis:

LIFESTYLE	If your lifestyle is complicated by mental stress or by smoking, then these will aggravate psoriasis. Self-help measures can help you break away from a vicious circle in which behaviour and psoriasis interact (see Chapters 3, 14, 15, 16).
ALLERGIES	Most people with psoriasis don't have an allergy that influences the rash. However, fashion jewellery may cause particular problems in young women. The relationship between metal allergy and psoriasis is not always recognised. This aspect is therefore discussed in detail in Chapter 18.
YEASTS	If there is a change in the normal balance of bacteria and yeasts living on the skin, the yeasts may provoke a response from the immune system. This worsens skin inflammation, especially in the scalp and the body folds. (Also see Chapters 6 and 8, and Appendix 3.)

KEY POINTS

- Self-help measures can play an important role in controlling psoriasis.

- Self-help should complement the medical treatment provided by your doctor.

2 THE PROBLEM AND THE AIMS

Practically everyone knows someone with psoriasis. It is estimated that at least 2% of the population of the UK have this problem. Many of these people are young.

A Simple Outline

Certain facts about this common condition are listed below:

1 Psoriasis is not catching.

2 It is a benign condition. There is no link between psoriasis and the risk of cancer.

3 Psoriasis runs in some families, but not everyone in the family develops it. What gets passed on is a tendency for it to appear. This

may not happen until someone is well into old age, or may not happen at all.

4   There is no easy method of predicting how temporary or troublesome it may become. Psoriasis remains mild in most people.

5   Psoriasis has several different phases of activity, as shown in the diagram below:

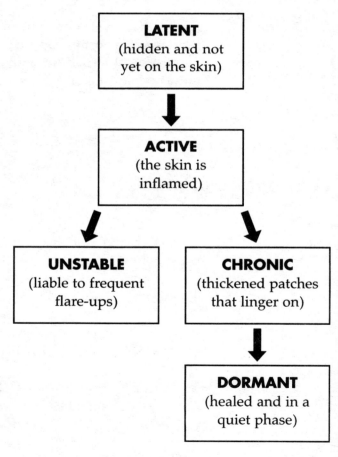

LATENT
(hidden and not yet on the skin)

↓

ACTIVE
(the skin is inflamed)

UNSTABLE
(liable to frequent flare-ups)

CHRONIC
(thickened patches that linger on)

↓

DORMANT
(healed and in a quiet phase)

Why Psoriasis appears

We don't know what causes psoriasis. What we do know is that psoriasis surfaces when certain types of injury to the skin produce a faulty healing response. It is believed that some people inherit the genes that give them a tendency to develop psoriasis.

Psoriasis appears on the skin because:

1 The inflamed skin has been injured. This injury may be mainly physical, mainly chemical from within the body, or a mixture of physical and chemical.

2 There has been a change in the delicate balance of the skin's immunity.

The sequence of changes is shown in the diagram below:

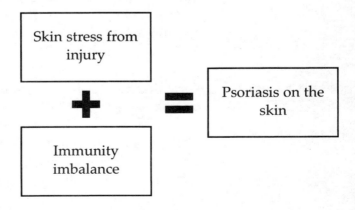

Skin Changes

When the skin is inflamed, extra blood is attracted to the area. This blood makes the skin appear red.

Psoriasis also causes another change to the skin. In healthy skin, dead cells from the skin's surface are shed in tiny invisible clumps. In skin affected by psoriasis, the dead surface layers of skin are shed as large white flakes.

As already explained, the skin changes typical of psoriasis occur when injury to the skin is followed by a faulty healing response from the immune system.

Skin Injury

Three common types of injuries – which often overlap – may cause psoriasis to appear on the skin surface.

KNOCKS AND STRETCHES

Normally, the skin can stand up to knocks, stretches and strains. However, if such injuries are persistent, then the response in some people is an area of psoriasis. This is why, for example, someone may develop psoriasis rather than a scar at the site of a cut.

INFECTION OF BODY FOLDS	Germs, such as bacteria and yeasts, collect easily in the body folds. There, the combination of warmth and humidity allows them to multiply particularly rapidly. As they live off the skin, and also when they die, the germs cause the skin to become inflamed. Next, moisture in the body folds softens the skin and allows it to split. A crack appears and the inflammation spreads. It is in this way that psoriasis can make the skin sore in body areas such as the buttock folds and under the breasts.
THROAT INFECTION	A throat infection sets off a chain reaction in the blood. Sometimes, this causes psoriasis to appear as tiny red dots like rain-drops on the trunk, arms and legs.

Skin Response

Our skin works as a whole. It should be thought of as a single organ. If one area of the skin is under stress, then so is the rest of it.

In someone with psoriasis, matters become more complicated. There is a fault in the skin's natural healing response. If the skin is severely provoked, the resulting inflammation may affect the skin over the entire body. Fortunately, this is a very rare event.

Patterns of Psoriasis

We don't know all the factors that influence how active or widespread the rash becomes.

The amount of injury the skin receives and the state of the immune system both affect the activity of psoriasis. However, we do not know what other factors may also play a part in keeping it in an active phase.

In most people, the psoriasis remains in a quiet phase for most of the time. Often, when psoriasis appears on the surface, the red patches are limited to the elbows and the knees. Sometimes, the scalp is the only inflamed area. In the vast majority of affected people, the condition doesn't progress beyond these areas. Only a few people have psoriasis that affects problem areas such as the hands and the feet.

Your Aim

The steps necessary to control the problem are:

1 Reduce skin injury.

2 Improve skin hygiene.

3   Attend to general health and thereby improve the immune system.

By following these steps, you can help check the full-blown responses of the skin that produce psoriasis. Various creams and tablets may heal the rash up to a point. Aim to hasten your recovery and to be rid of the rash for a long time. The detailed advice in the chapters that follow should help you achieve this goal.

KEY POINTS

- Psoriasis heals more quickly when attention is paid to skin care. Good skin hygiene is particularly important for people with psoriasis. Aim to maintain a high level of skin care and to make this a habit.

- It may be more difficult to keep up a good level of general health. However, if this is possible, you will benefit from having a more efficient immune defence system. This is one way of controlling the psoriasis.

3 *THE MENTAL APPROACH*

It is quite likely that you have heard how troublesome and disabling psoriasis can be. Your first reactions when the rash was diagnosed might have been:

- Why me?

- How will psoriasis affect my life?

- Will it be as bad as I have seen or heard it to be?

Ways of Coping

Different people respond in different ways. You may feel angry and resentful. These are frequent and understandable reactions.

You might then decide to tackle the problem by:

1 Learning to ignore it altogether. This method works for many people.

2 Relying mainly on the medical treatment and letting the condition rule your life. If you do this, psoriasis may limit you in all sorts of ways, especially in your social life.

3 Taking charge of the problem and arranging matters so that psoriasis is no more than a minor nuisance. This puts you – and not the condition – in control of your life.

Lifestyle Effects

A stressful life worsens many conditions in which the immune system plays an important role. Your psoriasis might have been triggered off by a stressful event. If, as a result, you feel guilty about it, then the problem is made worse. Try not to feel guilty.

Remember that there are excellent medical treatments that will help most people with psoriasis. A change of lifestyle can then help to keep the skin healed. It typically takes many months to achieve this benefit but it is well worth the effort.

An optimistic approach reverses the vicious circle of stress and misery that keeps the psoriasis in an active phase.

The Aim

Think of psoriasis as a particular type of reaction from the skin. Understand the factors that make it worse. Work out your own ways of limiting these injuries. Then, let your body's own healing mechanisms come into play.

Self-reliance

All the practical guidelines for treating psoriasis point in the direction of self-reliance. You may find that you are able to follow only some of the guidelines. Even then, you are helping your body to control the psoriasis.

Relying on yourself in this way may be easy for you. Your immune system may be in good shape and your body may shrug off the psoriasis easily. If not, you can still achieve much the same result if you follow the practical guidelines step by step.

If psoriasis is totally ignored as a problem, the stress it has caused diminishes. The immune system is then able to induce healing of the skin. This mental approach to psoriasis is difficult, but it may also prove satisfactory.

KEY POINTS

- It is possible to control this condition, especially if you tackle it head-on at an early stage. Simply relying on medical treatment may or may not work for you. The rash may keep on re-appearing despite the use of effective creams.

- As in many medical disorders, the right mental approach is all important. Be determined to suppress the psoriasis, even if there are set-backs.

4

IMMUNITY AND THE SKIN

The immune system has a significant influence on the changes in the skin which result in psoriasis. An understanding of the link between immunity and psoriasis is therefore important.

The Immune System and the Skin

Inflammation is the skin's normal response to injury. Healing then follows. Both these skin changes are controlled by our immunity.

If psoriasis is in its active phase, skin inflammation persists and the healing is not complete. (The different types of injury which provoke psoriasis are described in Chapter 2.)

When psoriasis is active, the skin's immune system doesn't function effectively. The skin's immune system is, of course, part and parcel of the whole body's immunity.

Immune Responses in Psoriasis

Our immune system has its own checks and balances. In psoriasis, these influence the skin in different ways. Immune responses affect:

1 How effectively a throat infection is overcome, and whether the skin responds to the infection, as it does in some people, by producing psoriasis.

2 How easily the inflammation in the skin is checked from appearing on the skin as psoriasis.

3 How quickly the skin on which psoriasis appears then heals to produce normal skin.

Immunity and Skin Healing

We don't know why all of the immune responses in psoriasis are not in balance. From time to time, these fail to check the inflammation in the skin. Healing may take a long time or prove to be temporary. The condition keeps flaring up.

There are many disorders in which our immunity develops a fault in its healing responses. It may over-react in some conditions or perform less well in others. Don't imagine that because you have psoriasis, you may develop any of these other conditions.

Lifestyle and Immunity

If your lifestyle is unhealthy, a change to a healthy lifestyle would obviously benefit your immunity. This is a slow process, however. The influence on psoriasis may not be apparent for many months.

It is of course possible to have mild psoriasis, limited to patches on the elbows or the knees, even with a healthy lifestyle. These may linger on as long as psoriasis remains in a chronic phase.

Influences on Immunity

A change in the normally delicate balance in the immune system will be a result of various influences. Many of these have yet to be fully understood. From a practical point of view, the important ones are:

1 A build-up of toxic chemicals in the body from tobacco smoking.

2 Mental stress.

Both of these influences are discussed in detail later in this book (Chapters 14 and 15).

KEY POINTS

- Our understanding of all the changes in the immune system that occur with psoriasis is limited. Only a small and subtle change may be keeping the condition active, especially in someone with mild psoriasis. Once the balance is restored, the skin heals and remains healed.

- If your general health is good, then so is your body's immunity. You may have difficulties in getting the balance completely in your favour. This is a common problem. Regard whatever you achieve as a positive step in gaining control over your psoriasis.

5 *GENERAL CARE OF THE SKIN*

Inflamed skin loses water easily and then dries out. It also cannot tolerate stretching in the same way as normal skin. If you have psoriasis you should treat your skin gently. This is the basis of the advice given in this chapter and in other parts of this book.

Local Skin Care

It is not advisable to pick off the scales from patches of psoriasis. Also, don't make a habit of picking at patches on the elbows.

Rubbing or scraping off the scales in psoriasis will only inflame the skin more. The white flakes on the surface of the patches will gradually vanish as the skin heals.

If an area becomes itchy, you can reduce the itch as follows:

1   Press down on the patch for a few minutes with a damp handkerchief.

2   Wet the patches with luke-warm salt water and then rub in Vaseline or a bland hand cream.

3   Air the room. Poor ventilation – of an office, for example – affects skin comfort. The room may have become too hot for the skin to be comfortable. The skin is also affected if the humidity is either too low or too high.

4   Change into loose comfortable clothes.

Reducing Local Injury

As a general rule, the skin in some areas of the body – such as the palms – can stand up to rough treatment. In someone with psoriasis, this ability is reduced. In fact, if the skin anywhere on the body is repeatedly stretched or rubbed – as commonly occurs at work – the response may well be an area of inflamed skin.

Aim to reduce the amount of stretching or rubbing which your skin suffers.

Baths

1   It is not necessary to have daily baths because you have psoriasis. In fact, after a few weeks, daily baths may make the skin dry all over. You might, however, find it helpful to soak affected areas daily before applying a cream that has been prescribed for you. Damp skin absorbs some drugs more easily.

2   If possible, have showers. If not, keep the bath time short and the water not too hot. Inflamed skin does not tolerate heat very well.

3   Use a simple non-medicated soap. Avoid scented products, especially if you are allergic to perfumes.

4   Don't scrub away at patches on areas such as the elbows and knees.

5   Always pat the skin dry, especially the inflamed areas. Be fussy. Don't leave the skin to dry off on its own. Inflamed skin left to dry off cools rapidly and is more liable to crack.

6   Dry all the body folds carefully, as a habit. Pay attention to the ear-folds, the armpits, the navel, under the breasts, the groin and the toe-webs.

7   At a swimming pool, apply Vaseline to any patches of psoriasis before you swim. If the chemicals added to the water still irritate the skin, then have a shower after the swim.

Cosmetics

If you have a perfume allergy, use hypoallergenic products that suit you. A wide range of scented products, from deodorants to fabric-softeners, may contain ingredients that are chemically related to those in perfumes.

If you are allergic to lanolin, select products labelled as free from lanolin.

If the skin in the armpit is inflamed, then use salt washes to dry it out. Once the rash has subsided, use non-scented deodorants if you are perfume sensitive.

Most department stores have staff who can advise on suitable masking creams for use on the hands or the face. Products that are waterproof are also available. You can, of course, apply your usual make-up without spreading the rash.

For hair removal, cold wax treatment is less damaging to the skin than the hot wax routine.

Weather Protection

Inflamed skin cannot put up with weather damage. Wrap up well for protection from cold strong winds. Use a scarf, hood and gloves if the face and hands are sore.

During a quiet phase, the skin affected by psoriasis may benefit from sunlight. However, if patches of psoriasis are red and raw, the skin is more likely to burn.

Patches on the Legs

Standing for long periods allows blood to pool in the legs. The veins in the legs may not always be efficient in returning the blood to the heart. The problem is worse if you are tall or overweight.

Leg veins swell long before they become varicose veins. There is, therefore, a back-pressure effect on the skin. The pressure stretches the skin from underneath. As a result, a weak spot of inflamed skin becomes weaker and stretches even more. (See colour plate at the centre of this book.)

Patches of psoriasis on the shins or the calves are often very itchy. The ankles may also swell at the end of the day. The pressure effects on the skin can be reduced in two ways:

1 Wear support bandages, tights or stockings during the day. Remember that bandages lose their stretch after several washes and need to be replaced.

2 Exercise the calf muscles by bending the legs at the knees from time to time. The muscles then pump the extra blood in the legs back to the heart.

KEY POINTS

- The skin acts as a barrier against a range of insults. These may be:
a) physical – knocks and stretching
b) chemical – such as detergents
c) atmospheric – strong winds or very bright sunlight.
Since the ability to tolerate these insults is diminished in psoriatic patches, you need to protect your skin.

- Once inflamed, the raw areas of the skin lose heat and water. By contrast, in the body folds, warmth and humidity allow germs to multiply. Don't let the inflamed skin become too dry or too moist for comfort.

- Whenever the skin is inflamed and sore, treat it gently.

6 CARE OF THE INFLAMED SCALP

It is a normal process for the scalp to shed clumps of generally invisible skin cells. However, an inflamed scalp produces larger quanties of more easily seen white flakes of skin cells. A sharp or steady pull on the hair, while combing or brushing, tugs at the roots and makes the problem of scalp inflammation worse.

Troublesome Areas

Scalp areas which often become inflamed are:

1 The nape of the neck and above the ears.

2 Behind the ears and the ear-folds.

3 On the forehead along the hair-line and also in the hair parting.

Triggers at different sites

Different trigger factors are involved at each of the scalp's three main trouble sites.

THE NAPE

A patch of psoriasis on the back of the head or behind the ear is often very itchy. It gets scratched and becomes worse. Scratching becomes a habit. At times of stress, the patch becomes the focal point for relieving anxiety by scratching. Aim to break this habit.

EAR-FOLDS

Little light or air may get to the deep fold behind the ears. If moisture builds up there, then the skin splits. Bacteria and yeast settle into the crack and worsen the condition.

HAIR-LINE AND
PARTING

Frequent and repeated pulling on the hair, as when combing or brushing, provokes more inflammation around the hair roots.

The strongest pulling usually occurs along the hair-line at the forehead, particularly when the hair is being combed back. Strong pulling of the hair, and inflammation of the follicles from which the hairs grow, is also common on either side of the parting. (See colour plates at the centre of the book.)

Hair Care

1 Always wash and dry the scalp gently. Don't try to scrub away scaly patches.

2 Don't use a nylon hair brush. Use a pure bristle or a mixed bristle and nylon one. Always comb and brush the hair gently.

3 When a brush or a comb is run all the way through the hair, the pull on the follicles along the parting increases. This injury keeps them inflamed. Pressing down with a finger, just beyond the parting (or above the hairline), reduces this strain. It is also important to brush the hair gently.

4 Avoid a hair style that requires the use of grips or clips. Also avoid hair bands that pull tightly on the hair.

5 When psoriasis on the scalp is particularly troublesome, a short hair style may be easier to manage.

6 The ear-folds must be kept dry. After a wash, use tissues to soak up the moisture. It may be advisable to alter the hair style to allow light and air to the area.

7 If the ear canal is inflamed, use cotton buds soaked in salt water to clean the area. Then

dry the ear canal. Don't prod. If the ears are clogged up, you need medical attention.

8 Don't use a medicated shampoo for months on end. From time to time, use a mild non-medicated shampoo. This allows the scalp to regain its normal balance of organisms.

9 Heated rollers and curlers cause pulling at the hair roots and damage the texture of the hair. When using a hair dryer, always keep it at least 30 cm (1 ft) away from the hair.

10 If the scalp is inflamed, postpone having a perm until the flaking is reduced. When you have a perm, warn the hairdresser about your psoriasis so that the treatment is kept gentle.

Matted Hair

If there is a heavy build up of scales on the scalp, the hair gets trapped in the scales and becomes matted. After treatment for psoriasis, the hair may be quite thin. As a rule, provided the problem is tackled at an early stage, any hair loss is only short term. The hair follicles will produce new hair.

Remember that a sensible healthy diet is important for good regrowth of hair.

Scalp Infection

If the scalp surface is broken, or the skin in the ear-folds is split, a sample from these areas may be sent for laboratory examination. Infection from bacteria can aggravate the inflammation.

If you are found to have a bacterial infection of the scalp, you will need suitable antibiotic treatment from your doctor.

KEY POINTS

- The white flakes in the scalp can cause much embarrassment. On the other hand, the hair often gets a great deal of unnecessary attention. This increases the risk of damage. Your hair does need to look good, but you should always treat the hair follicles gently. This rule applies even when the flaking has stopped.

- Repeatedly stretching the inflamed skin that supports the hair follicles is a physical injury that aggravates psoriasis.

- All scalp care must be gentle.

7 SKIN CARE FOR THE FACE

For cosmetic reasons, psoriasis on the face needs early attention. The aim is to suppress it and then take good care of the newly healed skin.

General Care

1 If you are using a hair style to hide red areas of psoriasis on the face, then you should let some light and air get to the skin whenever possible. Otherwise, a micro-climate is created that allows various germs to prolong the inflammation.

2 Always pat the skin dry after a wash.

3 Shaving may be easier with an electric shaver, at least until the redness has faded away and the new skin has hardened.

4 If psoriasis on the scalp and along the hair-line has spread down the forehead, then you should follow the advice on scalp care given in Chapter 6.

5 Sometimes there is a fine flaking of the skin in the eyebrows and the lashes. A luke-warm salt water wash for a couple of minutes 3 or 4 times a day may be enough to check the inflammation in this area.

6 Be certain as to how often and for how long you use a cream that has been prescribed for you, especially if it contains a cortico-steroid drug. It is important to have clear medical advice on this point.

7 A suitable camouflage or masking cream can be used while you are using a medicated cream to treat the rash.

8 The inflamed facial skin doesn't tolerate room conditions in which there is low humidity or poor ventilation. Obviously, you need expert advice if you cannot tackle the problem yourself.

9 Exposing the skin to chemical fumes and vapours at work could also aggravate the inflammation. You should talk to your employer about the possible arrangement of suitable extraction or humidification equipment that will allow you to work in a comfortable environment. A hobby may

cause you similar problems with fumes or vapours at home.

10 If your work or leisure activities involve contact with dirt or grease, you should take care not to transfer it to the face.

Weather Protection

When it is inflamed, the delicate facial skin is much more sensitive than usual to weather damage. It doesn't then adjust easily to temperature changes.

During autumn and winter, cold winds affect the skin in various ways. The skin is easily damaged by the force of the wind. Also, apart from buffeting the skin, the wind cools and dries the skin out. Before going outdoors, apply a face cream to reduce the drying effect of the wind. When you are out, wear a scarf or a hood.

In spring and summer, both heat and light rays from the sun can aggravate the inflammation. Always avoid direct strong sunlight so as not to burn the skin. If you are sun-sensitive, then use a suitable sunscreen (see Appendix 3). Otherwise, if you take care, gentle sunshine may help to heal the rash.

KEY POINTS

- When the facial skin is inflamed, the redness affects your confidence. It is important to treat the skin regularly with the cream that has been prescribed for you. At the same time, control the factors which aggravate the problem.

- It is not usual for psoriasis to spread all over the face. A rash on the face may have other explanations. Get expert advice to check on the diagnosis.

- Once inflamed, the skin doesn't tolerate the weather as well as it used to. Protect your face, so that the newly healed skin has a chance to toughen up.

8 SKIN CARE FOR BODY FOLDS

All the body folds collect moisture. Some of them, for example the armpits, are also sweat-producing areas. The circulation of air in body fold areas is often poor. As a result, the skin becomes warm and moist. These conditions make the body folds excellent places for yeasts and bacteria to settle and flourish in.

In this way, psoriasis may appear behind the ears, in the armpits, under the breasts and in the navel and the groin.

Aim to keep the skin folds as dry as possible. This rule applies even after the psoriasis has healed up.

General Care of Body Folds

Various aspects of general skin care, which also relate to the body folds, are discussed in

Chapter 5 of this book. Three of special note are listed here:

1 Wear loose comfortable clothing whenever possible. The best fabrics are cotton or cotton and polyester. Women should avoid wearing underwired bras as these encourage sweating.

2 Be fussy about drying body fold areas properly after a wash. Use paper tissues to get rid of the last traces of moisture.

3 Before using a cream that has been prescribed for you, bathe the area with luke-warm salt water for 5 to 10 minutes. Pat the skin dry and then rub in a thin smear of the cream. A few minutes later, wipe off any excess cream with tissues.

Split Skin

As the moisture in the skin itself increases, the skin softens. It then splits. A crack behind the ears, under the breasts or between the buttocks can be quite painful. It is also difficult to heal. The problem is worse if you are plump.

Certain actions at work can sometimes aggravate psoriasis. For example, a receptionist may hold a telephone receiver against the same ear many times during the day. The pressure from the receiver causes the skin fold behind that ear to soften and then split. Such splits are very prone to infection.

Any infection of splits in the skin can be checked for. A sample from the depth of the fold can be tested in a laboratory. If an infection is found, this complication needs antibiotic treatment.

Certain bacteria that are known to produce throat infections, and as result trigger off psoriasis, are also capable of infecting the body folds.

Skin Care of the Groin

1 Wear comfortable clean cotton underwear. Avoid tight-fitting jeans and trousers. Synthetic tights, especially those made of thick lycra, encourage sweating. Wear stockings or socks instead. For men, boxer shorts are better than Y-fronts at letting air circulate in the skin folds.

2 In hot summer months, a regular wash with salt water at the end of the day may prevent the problem from re-appearing.

3   If at work you sit at a desk for long periods, use a cushion covered with a natural fibre. Sitting on synthetic material encourages sweating. The same applies for car seats.

4   Practise wet-wiping. The skin around the anus traps many germs. Thorough cleansing of the inflamed skin is therefore very important when using the toilet. As a last step in wiping the skin, moisten some toilet paper. Fold the moistened paper and then hold it with layers of dry paper as you use it to clean the skin. Then use tissues as the final step to soak up the moisture. (Packs of pre-moistened toilet paper sometimes contain a preservative that can irritate the skin.)

Vaginal Discharge

A vaginal discharge can inflame psoriasis in the area. The most common cause is a yeast infection, such as thrush. It may also be caused by bacteria that infect the throat and trigger off psoriasis. If you have a discharge, follow the medical treatment that is recommended as well as instructions on personal and sexual hygiene.

KEY POINTS

- The skin in the body folds is thin. When saturated with moisture, it splits. Be fussy about keeping it dry.

- Don't let the folds collect sweat for long periods. The skin deep in the folds must be allowed to breathe.

- Even when psoriasis has healed, maintain a good standard of hygiene. The extra time spent on good hygiene habits will pay dividends.

9 SKIN CARE FOR THE HANDS

Psoriasis on the hands is a nuisance in two ways. It makes the hands difficult to use and its appearance causes embarrassment. The rash may be on the backs of the hands or mainly on the palms.

Backs of the Hands

There are two main types of injury to the skin in this area:

1 Sunlight: the sun's rays may aggravate the rash, especially if the skin on the face, neck and arms is also inflamed. The effects of sunlight on the skin are discussed in Chapter 11. A suitable camouflage cream can be used to mask the redness until the skin heals.

2 Stretching: frequent stretching of the knuckle joints keeps the skin inflamed. The red inflamed areas on the fingers may develop on the knuckles or on the skin between the knuckles. The injury can occur at home or at work. Friction on the skin anywhere on the hands also causes inflammation. (For information on how this type of injury to the hands can be reduced, see Chapter 19.)

Nail-folds and the Nails

The cuticle on each nail acts as a seal between the nail and the skin, thus protecting this area from infection and also from irritation from chemicals. After months of regular wet work, this protective barrier breaks down. The nail-fold becomes easily inflamed. In fact, it provides a pocket in which germs can flourish. Eventually, psoriasis appears around the nails.

Follow these skin care measures to look after your nails:

1 Don't pick at the cuticle as a habit, or destroy it during manicuring.

2 Your aim is to keep the nail-folds dry. Always dry each finger tip separately. Use tissues to soak up the moisture in the nail-folds. Take your time.

3 A sample from the swollen nail-folds can be checked for evidence of any infection. Your doctor can arrange the test.

4 If using a cream, apply it to the area sparingly. Wipe off any excess. It may sometimes be better to use a lotion instead of a cream to treat the infection (see Appendix 3).

5 Psoriasis in the nails distorts them, making them difficult to trim. Use nail clippers instead of scissors. Trim back the corners of the nails carefully. This is especially important when cutting toe-nails. Otherwise, the corners at either side grow into the flesh and inflame the skin.

6 Keep the nails short. A long finger-nail catches easily. The injury then inflames the bed from which the nail grows.

7 Use varnish to hide any distortions in the nail until it grows again normally. Using artificial nails will also help in hiding the defects.

8 Keep the finger-nails clean. The pocket under the ends of the nails allows yeasts and bacteria to shelter. These can be re-introduced to the skin whenever an inflamed area is

scratched. Using a cream that kills off this population of germs may be helpful (see Appendix 3).

The Palms

Once the hard skin on the palms becomes inflamed, it splits easily. The cracks let in germs. Then a vicious cycle of inflammation and infection is set up. (Sometimes it is a fungus infection, often by yeasts, that provokes the inflammation.)

In most people, the thick skin on the palms can stand up to both stretching and friction. Friction against the tender skin with psoriasis is difficult to avoid. This is another reason why the inflammation lingers on. The constant injury to the hands may occur at work, for example when a plumber uses wrenches or other tools in his job. At home, do-it-yourself jobs, or even a gentle repetitive activity such as knitting, can keep the psoriasis active.

One way of healing the cracks, is to seal the hand in a polythene glove or in a bag with a tape over the wrist. After a few hours, moisture builds up and the skin softens. This method can be used every evening until the cracks begin to heal.

Role of Allergies and Detergents

When a rash appears on the hands as a result of wet work at home, the skin problem is often called housewife's eczema. When skin damage is caused by frequent skin contact with chemicals at work, the problem is described as dermatitis. Someone with psoriasis is equally liable to run into both these problems.

Sometimes, an allergic reaction could trigger the psoriasis on the hands or keep it active. A metal allergy to nickel can show up as inflammation on the palms. Rubber gloves can cause a reaction to some of the chemicals they contain. Soaps and detergents, if frequently used, take away the natural oils from the skin. It then feels dry and cracks easily.

Quite often, these different types of skin injury combine together to make the psoriasis on the hands a chronic problem.

Hand Care

Follow the skin care advice given here in addition to the treatment that your doctor prescribes for you.

GLOVES

For wet jobs, use thin cotton gloves with unlined vinyl gloves on top. The cotton gloves can be rinsed out in case some detergent has seeped in. Wear cotton gloves when dusting.

At work, use the gloves specially provided for the job. Aim to avoid skin contact with oil, grease and other chemicals. Wear the gloves as a matter of habit and change them often. If they make the hands sweat, wear thin cotton gloves underneath. Cutting off the tips of the fingers of the gloves may make it easier to do delicate jobs. In the winter, protect the skin from cold air by wearing woollen or leather gloves.

DRYING THE SKIN

Some areas of the skin can collect moisture if they are not properly dried. These include the finger-webs, the nail folds and under any rings. Be fussy and use tissues as the final step. Regular use of a hand cream that suits you is one way of coping with the injury caused by soaps and detergents.

REST FROM INJURY

The inflamed skin has to heal before it is tough enough to stand up to all the knocks of daily living. It can be very difficult to organise your life to make this possible. At this stage, you may well need support from your family.

KEY POINTS

- Most people with psoriasis don't get the rash on the hands. There is, however, a limit to the amount of damage from chemicals our skin can tolerate. Don't wait until that limit of tolerance is reached. Good hand care is important, be it at home or at work.

- Psoriasis on the hands is a frustrating experience and is sometimes a disability. Occasionally allergies can involve the skin on the hands. This is a complex problem for which you need expert advice.

- Even with regular treatment with creams and with good skin care, it may take months for the psoriasis to heal. When it is healed, maintain the same level of skin care so that the problem doesn't re-appear.

10 SKIN CARE FOR THE FEET

The pattern of psoriasis on the feet depends on the site of injury to the skin. It may be mostly on the toes, on the soles or on top of the feet.

Weight Bearing Areas

The hard skin on the soles protects the deeper lying arteries, nerves and muscles. It also bears the body's weight. This load is shared equally between the heels and the toes, with the instep acting as an arch.

When inflamed, the skin on the heels and under the toes produces a thick layer of dead skin of poor quality. As a result, the skin splits and the feet become sore. The cracks allow germs an easy entry and the inflammation spreads. (See colour plate at the centre of the book.)

The problem is worse if you are tall, heavy and stand a lot at work, or have fallen arches and flat feet. Activities such as jogging or aerobics obviously add insult to injury.

Sometimes, if the leg veins are swollen, the tiny blood vessels under the insteps also swell (see Chapter 5.) The back-pressure stretches the skin and psoriasis may appear on the insteps.

Inflamed Soles

In addition to the treatment prescribed for you, the following measures should help:

1 When the condition is active, soak the feet in luke-warm salt water for about 10 minutes, three times a day. During the soak, separate the toes so that all the skin in the webs comes in contact with the salt water. Afterwards, pat the skin dry carefully. During hot summer months, salt water soaks every night may prevent psoriasis from re-appearing.

2 Any cream prescribed for you should be rubbed in sparingly and the excess wiped off after about 10 minutes.

3 Quite often the skin on the heels dries out and splits. Sealing the foot in a polythene bag

with a tape across the ankle, for a few hours in the evening, may help to soften the skin and heal the cracks.

4 If the ankles tend to swell at the end of the day, follow the advice on support bandages given in Chapter 5.

5 In the winter months, keep the feet warm. This is important, especially if the circulation of blood in the legs is poor and the feet tend to be cold.

Footwear

1 All footwear should be light-weight and comfortable. Fashionable shoes with pointed toes damage the growing bones and skin, especially in young children. Shoes with leather soles absorb moisture. Synthetic shoes don't soak up sweat or let the skin breathe.

2 When the skin is inflamed, choose insoles that relieve the pressure on the skin. These may be of padded foam, cork or water-filled. To protect newly healed skin, shock-absorbent insoles made of a polymer are also available. These insoles should be worn with good quality running shoes. Trainers which are

soft and made of fabric that allows the sweat to evaporate may be suitable.

3 Avoid any socks that are mostly synthetic. The same applies to tights and stockings, especially during the summer months.

Role of Allergies

An allergy to some of the chemicals in footwear could set off psoriasis or keep it active (see Chapter 17). A red patch may appear under a shoe buckle because of metal allergy. Rubber chemicals or chrome salts in leather shoes can trigger off an allergic reaction. The rash is mainly on top of the toes and where the shoe insoles touch the skin under the feet.

Toe-webs and Nails

In someone with psoriasis, athlete's foot needs suitable treatment for the infection. When the skin between the toes remains moist, this micro-climate encourages fungi and bacteria to grow.

The infection then spreads around the toes and can also involve the toe-nails.

Aim to keep these areas dry. After a wash, always dry the skin between each of the toes properly. Use tissues to clean away dirt and sweat from the cracks deep in the folds. Don't let the skin here become white and sodden, especially under the little toe.

Toe-nails grow faster in people with psoriasis and need regular trimming. Use nail clippers and make sure the corners at the end of the nails are cut back as well. Otherwise, the edges of the nails keep on growing and dig deep into the skin. If you use scissors, cut the nails in a curve, using the base of the scissors where the blades meet.

Care of Healed Skin

Once the inflammation of psoriasis dies down, the skin on the soles stops producing a lot of hard white flakes. It is still red but quite thin. It now has to be allowed gradually to become as tough as it once was. The skin must not become too dry or too wet. This is a difficult balance to maintain but is critical for good skin care.

KEY POINTS

- Sore feet with painful cracks cause a lot of misery. Work hard at taking care of the healed skin. The aim is to avoid the cycle in which injury perpetuates inflammation.

- Creams and lotions can only partially check the inflammation, especially in the summer months. Good daily hygiene is also very important.

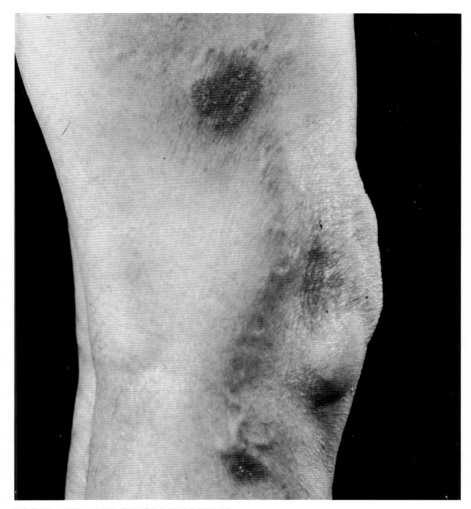

PSORIASIS AND SWOLLEN VEINS

The common problem of swollen veins on the legs aggravating psoriasis is easily overlooked. Standing still for a few minutes makes these veins prominent. Otherwise, they are faint blue lines and not seen as related to the patches of psoriasis. The steady back-pressure first stretches the skin and then inflames it. This persistent injury may keep the rash elsewhere on the body in an active stage, since the skin responds as a single organ.

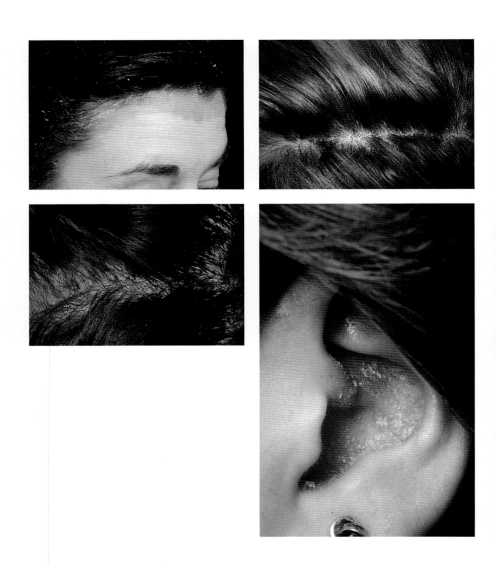

PSORIASIS IN THE SCALP

Psoriasis is common along the hair-line (*top left*) and parting (*top right*). Injury during brushing causes redness and flaking. Gradually, scales build up and the hair becomes matted (*above left*). Psoriasis in the ear (*above right*) usually responds well to treatment but may reappear unless the hair-style allows light and air to reach the area.

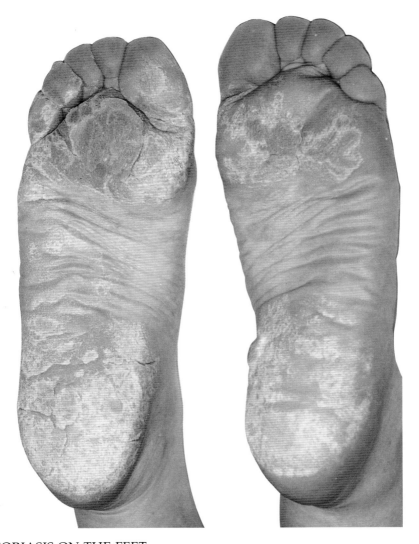

PSORIASIS ON THE FEET

When we walk, a pressure of one and a quarter times the body's weight is placed on each foot. This pressure is distributed between the heel, the ball of the foot and the underside of the little toe. These high-pressure areas are the parts of the foot most often affected by psoriasis. Treatment should include the use of arch supports and shock-absorbing insoles.

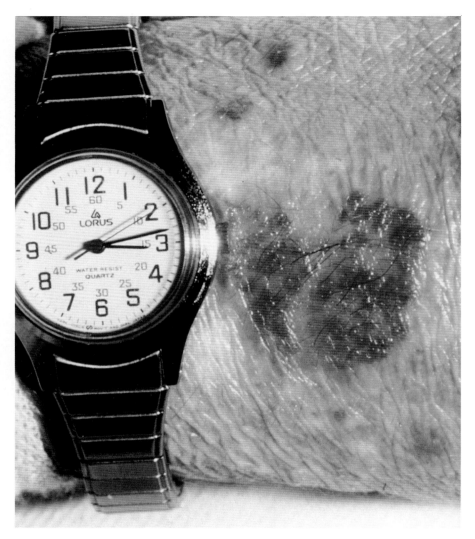

METAL-RELATED PSORIASIS

A tightly worn watch can aggravate psoriasis. Sweat leaches out nickel wherever the metal parts of the watch are in close contact with the skin. The result is skin inflammation, which is made worse by friction. It would be sensible to avoid wearing a watch with metal parts until the skin is healed.

11 *SUNLIGHT AND SKIN CARE*

Our skin responds to sunlight in a complicated way. Exposing the skin to sunlight is a highly effective method of suppressing psoriasis. Selected bands of ultra-violet light are, therefore, used in hospital clinics to treat psoriasis with dramatic effect.

Sunlight can influence psoriasis in various ways:

1 It may hasten healing and keep the psoriasis in a dormant phase.

2 In some people who can't tolerate sunlight, the condition remains active.

3 It can burn the skin and make the psoriasis worse.

Sunlight and Healing

1 Gentle and gradual sunbathing is of benefit to most people with psoriasis. However, you also need to follow the advice on skin protection given later in this chapter. Regard sunlight as a type of radiation hitting the skin. Use it therefore with care and in moderation. Don't let the sun burn the skin.

2 Artificial sunlight treatment, carried out by trained staff in hospital clinics, is also effective. If you are using a sunbed for this purpose, then let your doctor know. This method is not as safe as it may appear to be.

Sun-sensitivity

In some people with psoriasis, the rash shows up mainly on the backs of the hands, the neck and the face. In women, it may also appear on the legs below the knees. These are areas of the skin that catch the sunlight. There are two main reasons for this response from the skin:

1 Some people with red hair and fair or freckled skin, or with fair skin and blue eyes,

cannot tolerate bright sunlight. Psoriasis is then most troublesome over the areas of the skin that receive most light.

2 Certain drugs, especially those used for treating high blood pressure or taken as water tablets (diuretics) can make the skin sensitive to sunlight. You should discuss this possibility with your doctor.

Sunburn and Psoriasis

Over the years, the risk of sunburn has increased, even in the UK. Both the heat and light rays of the sun can severely inflame the red patches. There will be two consequences:

1 As a result of this physical injury, psoriasis may spread and become more active.

2 Following a sunburn, certain types of skin cells don't always regrow in an orderly fashion. Some years later, they may surface as skin cancer. This risk applies to all of us.

Protection from Sunlight

Whether your skin is fair or not, and whatever the effects of sunlight on it, you need to protect your skin from sun injury. It is easy to burn the skin accidentally, especially during hot summer months.

Some general rules on skin care in the sun should be followed:

1   After a dark winter, our skin needs time to toughen up before it can tolerate bright spring sunlight. Take care to expose the skin only gradually.

2   Use a suitable sunscreen routinely – even if it does not seem very sunny. This is especially important if you are sun-sensitive.

3   Never sunbathe at mid-day.

4   Protect the scalp and the face from sunlight with a wide-brimmed hat.

5   The sand, sea and snow can all reflect a lot of light onto the skin. The sun's radiation – even indoors near a large window – can injure the skin.

6   Denim clothes are more effective than thin cotton ones at screening out the harmful rays of the sun.

7 Children who have psoriasis can easily be accidentally sunburned. A suitable sunscreen should be used routinely during the spring and summer months. The child should also wear a sun hat.

Holidays

Regular holidays are important in controlling psoriasis. The skin benefits both from the release of stress and from sensible sunbathing. Follow these guide-lines when you go away:

1 Take an ample supply of the cream you use and keep it in a cool place.

2 Pack a portable vacuum cleaner if the skin is very scaly. Shedding a lot of skin in a hotel bedroom could be embarrassing.

3 The red patches are liable to dry out in sunny weather. Use a moisturiser cream regularly.

4 If you are travelling to a tropical country, you may be advised to take tablets that reduce the risk of getting malaria. Some of these drugs make psoriasis worse. Discuss the choice of anti-malarial drugs with your doctor.

KEY POINTS

- Sunlight has a subtle effect on our immunity. It dampens the over-active inflammation in the skin. However, don't rely on this benefit as the only method of controlling the rash. Maintenance of a healthy immune system and close attention to skin care remain important.

- Sunburn aggravates psoriasis. A sunburn, or many years of exposure to bright sunlight, also increases the risk of skin cancer. Treat sunlight (real or artificial) with respect so that you get the most out of it without taking unnecessary risks.

12 PSORIASIS IN CHILDREN

Psoriasis in children most often takes one of the following forms:

- It is limited to the elbows and knees or to the scalp, and typically lingers on.

- Crops of tiny red dots cover the body from time to time, and then vanish after a few weeks.

In either case, the psoriasis becomes a major cosmetic nuisance to the child. The rash is often a cause of great embarrassment and may produce much quiet suffering. Teasing by other children can make the problem worse.

If a child has psoriasis, it is particularly important to take all possible steps to clear the rash. This chapter concentrates on some practical guide-lines that relate particularly to children with psoriasis.

Help for Children

1 Get expert medical attention and treatment for the child at an early stage. Carefully follow any medical advice that is given. Remember to apply regularly any creams that are prescribed. Keep up with this regime until the rash has cleared completely.

2 Encourage exercise and sport, but keep the activities varied. Aim not to let the same area of the skin be stretched repeatedly. Psoriasis may surface if the skin is stretched beyond the limit it can tolerate – as may occur, for example, with too much cycling.

3 Visits to the swimming pool don't have to be restricted. A rub of Vaseline on the sore areas before the dip may reduce any irritation from chemicals added to the water. Remember to carefully pat the affected areas dry afterwards.

4 If the feet are involved, then follow the specific advice given in Chapter 10. The skin has to be treated gently until it recovers. Avoid fashion footwear that is unsuitable for the skin. Once the psoriasis has been controlled, relax the rules from time to time.

5 An overweight child may be troubled with psoriasis in the skin folds or in skin stretch areas. Don't allow over-eating to compensate for any misery produced by psoriasis.

6 Maintaining the immune system in good shape is important. A child's immune system, like the rest of the body, is immature. A good balanced diet is especially important. Also, because smoking affects the immunity, the child must not be forced to be a passive smoker, breathing in air filled with other people's tobacco smoke. (Nor should he or she become an active smoker.)

7 The child obviously needs to be given support, love and re-assurance as often as possible. Don't, however, let the rash be used to manipulate you. Your aim is to teach your child not to regard psoriasis as a handicap. Attention to appearance and general grooming also helps to build up the child's self-confidence.

8 Teasing about the rash at school can be a serious problem. The child has to learn how to ignore hurtful remarks. The teasing will then usually stop. Discussion with the teacher, involving the child as well as his or her best friend, can be useful.

9 Mental stress – with various possible causes, either at home or at school – can affect the way the affected skin behaves. If the psoriasis becomes more active, thus increasing the distress, then expert help should be sought at an early stage.

KEY POINTS

- Early and detailed attention to treatment is very important in children. All the relevant advice on skin care has to be followed as strictly as possible.

- A sensible healthy diet is a necessity if the immature immune system is to be expected to overcome the psoriasis.

- The rash can become a serious cosmetic problem to a child. The young mind has to learn how to deal with it and how to suppress the psoriasis. The child therefore needs plenty of family support and guidance.

13 *FAMILY MATTERS*

This chapter looks at various ways that psoriasis can affect family life.

Psoriasis and inheritance

If you are thinking about having children, don't let the possibility that they could inherit psoriasis stop you. Psoriasis does not always run in families. Even when it does run in a family, all that is passed on – and then only to some members of the next generation – is an increased chance that psoriasis may develop at some time.

If you have psoriasis and your child then develops it, try not to feel guilty. Give him or her the best possible care (see Chapter 12). Also, don't imagine that your child's condition is bound to be as troublesome as your own.

Family Support

Living with someone who has psoriasis can be stressful for all concerned. Sometimes, the reason for the tension in the family is not even recognised. The general guide-lines given below may be helpful. You must, however, think carefully of the consequences of following such advice. The aim is to ease family tension and not to make it worse.

1 Anyone with psoriasis, especially when it is a cosmetic nuisance, needs extra support at home. The heart of the problem is often that failed social contacts cause feelings of rejection. Such feelings need to be discussed. The aim is to secure some understanding of these emotions.

2 The cosmetic aspect of psoriasis can be especially difficult for a teenager. A common teenage response is to behave in ways that the parents find difficult. This is often easier than asking for parental help. Parents should be aware of their child's need for support at this time.

3 Don't use your psoriasis to gain an advantage within the family or when among friends. This ploy might work some of the time. However, you may then find that sympathy is not there when you really need it.

4 It may help if the family can accept that a major upset aggravates psoriasis. Mental stress can trigger off an attack or keep psoriasis in an unstable state.

5 Intimate skin contact during sex becomes a problem when psoriasis is active. The sensitive skin in the groin is extremely uncomfortable when inflamed. Discussing these difficulties with your partner should prevent misunderstanding.

Female Hormones and Psoriasis

Hormonal changes in women have an effect on the skin and can influence psoriasis.

PERIODS

If pre-menstrual tension makes the psoriasis worse, you should seek medical advice. During a menstrual period, the psoriasis may worsen for the following reasons:

1 Female hormones alter the skin's immunity.

2 The skin is stretched slightly by the build-up of fluid in certain parts of the body such as the abdomen.

3 Mood changes indirectly affect the skin.

THE PILL	The pill doesn't have a clear-cut effect on the way psoriasis behaves in most women.
PREGNANCY	During pregnancy, your psoriasis could get better or remain much the same. As you gain weight, take extra care of the body folds to prevent a build-up of moisture in these areas.
MENOPAUSE	Seek medical advice if mental stress during the menopause seems to worsen the psoriasis. Hormone replacement therapy (HRT) doesn't seem to influence the rash.

KEY POINTS

- Try not to let psoriasis interfere with your enjoyment of family life.

- Family support can make a lot of difference to your efforts in checking the condition. However, be willing to work hard at gaining this advantage.

- When appropriate, be prepared to discuss with other family members the difficulties that psoriasis may cause you. This will help them give you a cushion of support at home.

14 *STRESS AND THE SKIN*

Mental stress has a strong influence on how active the psoriasis becomes. Psoriasis itself adds to the stress. Your aim is to get out of the cycle in which stress leads to psoriasis which then leads to further stress.

Types of Stress

Two types of stress can affect psoriasis:

1 A sudden shock, such as a road traffic accident, can make psoriasis active.

2 When there is longer-term mental strain, as for example in a divorce, psoriasis may be the body's weak spot. It either keeps flaring up, or responds poorly to treatment.

The Mechanism

Stress triggers a release of chemicals in the blood. As well as reaching other organs in the body, such as the heart, these chemicals also reach the skin. There are two consequences if the chemicals keep on being released:

1   Certain nerves in the skin become overactive. The skin then becomes easily inflamed.

2   The body's immunity is lowered. It can't then check the inflammation in the skin.

Habitual Scratching

It is a very common habit for people to keep scratching the same areas of skin as a method of relieving anxiety. The skin may respond to the repeated damage by producing a stubborn patch of psoriasis.

Favourite scratch areas in women are the nape of the neck, the elbows and around the waist-line above the hips. Men under stress tend to scratch the scalp above the ears, the middle of the chest and under the tops of the socks. Sometimes, in people of both sexes, the finger-nails and the folds of skin in the groins are damaged by repeated scratching.

The injured skin becomes itchy. The injury from scratching then inflames the skin even more. Obviously, to break this vicious circle you have to learn to relax.

Changes in Lifestyle

There are three important steps involved:

1 Recognise the fact that you are under stress.

2 Whether they occur at home or at work, identify your main problems.

3 While trying to resolve your difficulties, learn how to release your anxieties.

You may find useful advice in magazines, which often include articles on stress management. Alternatively, find a book that offers detailed and clear advice. To be useful, the advice has to be of a type that suits your lifestyle. Simple relaxation exercises, yoga and hypnotherapy are just some of the methods that can help the skin to recover.

General Advice

Some simple guide-lines on coping with stress in relation to the skin are set out below:

1 Work out a plan and then proceed with it step-by-step.

2 Be patient. It takes time for the skin to benefit from lifting the strain on the immune system.

3 It is important that you have enough sleep. When psoriasis is active, the skin needs to rest so that it can heal.

4 Allow for a short period of 5 or 10 minutes of breathing exercises (or meditation) both in the morning and before going to bed. This is a slow but simple method of not letting daily tensions influence the skin.

5 Don't stop trying to release your anxieties, even if one set of problems is followed by another. Aim to take charge of events as far as practical. You then also begin to control the psoriasis. Even partial success counts.

6 As the rash improves, so does the mental state. The strain from the immune system is then lifted. This means that it can now check the inflammation in the skin.

Alcohol and Stress

Alcohol breaks down in the body to release toxic chemicals. The skin is, of course, at the receiving end of the alcohol that builds up in the blood. This can make psoriasis worse in several ways :

1 The flushing of the skin that alcohol produces may aggravate the inflamed skin patches in some people.

2 In the longer term, the calories in alcoholic drinks may increase the body weight. People who are overweight have deep body folds which are often prone to psoriasis.

3 Drinking alcohol flushes out zinc in the urine. Zinc is an element which is needed by the body for the skin to heal quickly.

4 Any liver damage adds to the side-effects of some tablets used in treating psoriasis. This is especially relevant if you are prescribed methotrexate tablets.

Don't rely on alcohol to ease mental stress. Gradually limit what you drink. Regard alcohol as an occasional social pleasure. However, if you are addicted, then you need medical advice.

KEY POINTS

- In someone with psoriasis, long-term stress can be compared with persistent physical stretching of the skin. As you learn to unwind, you begin to control the problem.

- Changing your lifestyle can be a slow and difficult method of suppressing psoriasis. On the other hand, relaxation techniques don't have to be complicated. Stick to one that suits you and be patient.

- Don't rely on drugs (such as tobacco and alcohol) to ease your anxieties. The aim is not to live with your psoriasis, but make it slip into a quiet phase. Just a small effort may be enough to achieve this result.

15 *SMOKING AND IMMUNITY*

Our immunity guides the body's healing responses. These responses are less effective than usual in people who have psoriasis (see Chapter 4). The problem is made worse by smoking, which itself can cause a lowered level of immunity.

Activity of Psoriasis

Psoriasis has a wide range of activity. It can easily fluctuate from a dormant state to an unstable one (see Chapter 2). The rash is more likely to appear when the immunity is dampened. It is also noticeably more difficult to control in people who smoke.

Smoking and the Skin

There are thousands of different chemicals in a tobacco leaf. These include insecticides as well as the leaf's own constituent chemicals. Toxic tobacco chemicals easily enter the blood by way of the lungs. They are then carried to the body organs, including the skin. The skin is capable of handling only some of these chemicals.

Exposure to chemicals from smoking is not limited to people who are themselves smokers. Anyone who breathes in air filled with tobacco smoke takes the chemicals into their body. Such passive smoking can happen at home or at work.

Smoking and Psoriasis

Smoking makes psoriasis worse in various ways:

1 The immune defence system becomes less effective.

2 Smoking allows frequent throat infections due to viruses and bacteria. Some of these infections trigger attacks of psoriasis even if a sore throat is not noticed.

3 The toxic chemicals in the blood may interfere with the normal healing responses of the skin.

The body's own natural healing methods are important in helping to clear psoriasis.

Relaxation and Immunity

Some people can stop smoking with little difficulty. Others may be helped by hypnotherapy or by tapes available from "Well Woman" or similar clinics.

If you have found it difficult to give up smoking, one way is to learn a relaxation method for coping with stress (see also Chapter 14). The benefits of this method are:

1 As mental stress decreases, the psoriasis improves.

2 Gradually you won't find it necessary to smoke.

3 Once the habit of smoking is broken, then psoriasis comes under your control.

4 If giving up smoking is a choice you have made, then you are less likely to smoke again.

KEY POINTS

- Many young people with psoriasis fit the following description. Their psoriasis is in an active state. They suffer from the strain of working hard outside the home while bringing up a young family. They also smoke.

- It is easier to stop smoking if you first establish a habit of daily relaxation. Psoriasis will then be far less of a nuisance. Your self-confidence will improve. Once you reach this stage, you will be more capable of coping with stress and will feel less need to smoke.

16 DIET, WEIGHT AND EXERCISE

There is no diet that suppresses psoriasis. However, there are two very important reasons why you should eat sensibly. One is to avoid becoming overweight. The other is to provide your skin with all the vitamins and other nutrients it needs.

The Influence of Weight Gain

Several complications can result from carrying extra weight :

1 A large deposit of fat under the skin causes the skin to become stretched. Psoriasis may then appear over the stretched areas, such as around the waist-line.

2 Extra fat in body folds, such as in the armpits, under the breasts and in the groins, traps more moisture. The increased humidity encourages various germs to grow in the depths of the folds.

3 The joints, especially the hips, the knees and the joints in the feet, are put under stress by the need to carry extra weight. Eventually, these joints may become painful.

4 The veins in the legs may swell out. This causes back-pressure on the skin, which aggravates the psoriasis.

5 The skin on the soles of the feet has to bear the total body weight. As a result, the skin in these areas may split and become raw, especially over the pressure points, such as the heels and the toes.

Feeding the Skin

Just like all the other organs in the body, the skin needs a good supply of vitamins and minerals if it is to remain healthy. However, if there is a general shortage of these nutrients, the body as a whole tends to treat the skin as a poor relation.

A diet consisting mainly of burgers, chips, chocolate bars and low calorie drinks doesn't feed the immune system properly. You should eat a sensible and balanced diet that contains good supplies of fruit, vegetables and fibre. Guide-lines for healthy eating can be found in numerous magazine articles and popular health books.

If you are a strict vegetarian, you may be missing out on two important minerals. One is iron and the other is zinc. Check with your doctor if you think this could be the case. The skin needs both of them.

Exercise

Exercise benefits the immune system. For many other reasons, it makes sense to be both fit and supple. Once again, moderation is important. If you have always kept fit, then no special rules apply. If not, then don't take up vigorous exercise without some thought. You may need medical advice. Proceed gently. Pounding the pavements while jogging is hard on the knees and the feet. Gentle stretching of the body, as in yoga exercises, is the best way of remaining supple.

KEY POINTS

- You need a balanced diet to keep the immune system working in your favour.

- Don't starve the body. If you plan to lose weight, do so gradually. Also, don't swing to the other extreme. Don't allow yourself to build up layers of fat.

- Take exercise, but with care, especially if exercising is not already a habit.

17 *THE RELEVANCE OF ALLERGY*

Someone who has psoriasis may well develop an allergic reaction in the skin. The reaction may be the result of direct skin contact with a trigger substance. It may also be an expression on the skin of a wider allergic response from the body. In either case, the allergy may keep psoriasis in the active stage, especially if the reaction persists.

The whole of the skin can be involved in an allergic response. The same is also true of the skin's ability to produce psoriasis.

An Allergic Reaction

In an allergic reaction, a chemical provokes a response from our immune system. Even a tiny quantity of a chemical may have an effect. The result is inflammation of the skin.

The factors which influence how troublesome an allergic reaction becomes are:

1 The total amount of the chemical that has set off the chain reaction.

2 How sensitive the immune system is to the trigger at the time of the challenge.

3 How efficient the system is in checking the allergic response.

Recognising an Allergy

Proving an allergy in anyone is a complicated and sometimes unsatisfactory exercise. Some skin tests and blood tests can produce useful information. However, the interpretation of these results and the giving of appropriate advice needs both skill and experience.

To recognise an allergy, it is necessary to relate the skin's reaction very carefully to possible triggers. For example, does the skin react when you wear certain cosmetics or jewellery? If you suspect that you have a food allergy, it may help to keep a diary of what you eat. You should discuss your allergy problems with your medical adviser.

Common Skin Allergies

Some groups of items that commonly cause allergies are described below:

COSMETICS

The allergy may be to chemicals in perfumes, to lanolin or to other components added to the mixture. Proving which chemical in the cosmetic is the responsible one is sometimes difficult. You may need expert advice. In any case, it may be sensible to use bland products that suit your skin.

METAL COMPOUNDS

Some people have an allergy to chrome salts. These are used in tanning leather. Gloves and shoes made of leather tanned in this way can produce an allergic reaction on the hands and feet. Building cement also contains chrome salts. Another metal that causes allergy is nickel (see Chapter 18).

RUBBER COMPOUNDS

Rubber gloves and shoes with rubber soles contain chemicals to which the skin may become allergic. Sometimes the skin on the palms reacts in sympathy with the skin on the soles. Psoriasis on the feet can be triggered off by rubber chemicals, by dyes or by adhesives used in making shoes.

Other Skin Responses

DRUGS

Some drugs make psoriasis worse while others superimpose an allergic reaction on the skin. The medicines may have been prescribed for heart disease or high blood pressure (e.g., water tablets or diuretics) or for depression. Some antimalarial tablets also cause problems. Discuss the possibility of a drug reaction with your doctor.

FOOD

Some foods can cause an allergic skin response. There is no special allergy diet for anyone with psoriasis. However, if you know that you are allergic to a particular food, such as shellfish, it is sensible to avoid it.

If a wheat allergy has been proven, then the skin will obviously benefit once a suitable diet has been adopted.

Sometimes the allergic reaction is due not to the food itself, but to drugs that have got into the food. For example, there may be penicillin in the meat and dairy products in your diet.

There are also some food items which inflame the skin although no allergy is involved. Well-known examples are alcohol and hot spicy foods, both of which produce flushing of the skin.

General Advice

1   In a skin allergy, very tiny quantities of chemicals unleash a strong response from the skin. Follow all the advice in this chapter, at least until the problem is controlled.

2   Most people with psoriasis do not have an allergy that influences the rash. Besides, the science of allergy in relation to psoriasis is far from clear. There are many special clinics which claim to investigate allergies. They may well disappoint you. In any case, before starting on any strict diets, you should ask your doctor for advice.

KEY POINTS

•   If the skin is at the receiving end of an allergic reaction, then in someone with psoriasis, the problem is made worse.

•   Many factors shape the allergic responses from the skin. Identifying your allergy and relating it to your way of life can be quite difficult. On the other hand, most people with psoriasis do not have a food or skin allergy.

18 *METAL-RELATED PSORIASIS*

Allergic reactions related to metal are the commonest of all skin allergies. About 15% of all women in the UK are nickel sensitive. This allergy could be especially important to young women with psoriasis.

Psoriasis and Metal Contact

Metal allergy has been researched in great detail, but not in relation to psoriasis. Most cheap metal objects contain nickel, and it is this element which commonly leads to an allergy.

Close contact of nickel with the skin, together with sweating, releases nickel into the skin and then into the blood. A reaction may appear at the contact site, such as under a bra-hook. It may also occur in areas where sweat is eliminated from the body, such as on the palms.

The Evolution of Metal Allergy

The problem may appear after ear-piercing. A combination of wet work and frequent metal contact speeds up the process. Certain jobs, such as being a hair-dresser or a cashier, increase the risk of metal allergy.

In someone with psoriasis, tiny red dots may appear under the metal parts of the bra, under jeans studs and under belt or shoe buckles. The ear-lobes may remain inflamed after wearing ear-rings. Sometimes the rash is under a watch or where the metal parts in the strap rub against the skin (see colour plate at the centre of the book). Psoriasis in these areas may be due to friction or an irritant reaction. No allergy may be involved. Also, skin tests used to prove allergy are not always accurate in people with psoriasis.

Nickel Avoidance

A few simple measures can help to reduce close skin contact with metal objects.

CLOTHING   Choose underwear without metal fastenings. Don't wear fashion jewellery even for a few hours. Nickel-free fashion jewellery is now available. Change to a watch with a plastic strap and wear it loose. You can also paint the metal parts in clothes, jewellery and watches with a special varnish sold by pharmacists or jewellers (see Appendix 3).

DIET

Some items in the diet can increase the nickel levels in the blood. Among them are tinned foods, drinks from vending machines, chocolates and related items, nuts, oats and liquorice. Avoid eating such items, especially chocolates, on an empty stomach.

KEY POINTS

- If you do have nickel allergy, direct skin contact with only a tiny amount of nickel can provoke inflammation. When such a reaction occurs in the blood, all of the skin is at the receiving end. The patches of psoriasis are, of course, included in this response.

- Not all metal-related reactions are allergic in origin. Nickel can irritate the skin and add to the inflammation. You may not have an allergy to this metal. However, the advice on avoiding close skin contact with metal objects is not usually difficult to follow.

19 *CARE OF THE JOINTS*

A very small group of people who have psoriasis are liable to have inflamed joints. The affected joints are often those in the fingers and the wrists. In some people, a large joint such as the ankle may swell up. This is followed some time later by the appearance of psoriasis on the skin.

The main reason for the inflammation is the strain that is put on the same joint many times during the day.

Patterns of Joint Strain

Like the skin, joint tissues can't stand up to a lot of stretching. Some examples of how joints can be strained are described here:

1   The strain may be due to a push and pull action on the finger and thumb joints. An

electrician, plumber or bus driver, for example, would put quite a strain on these joints day after day.

2   A bank cashier is more likely to damage the finger joints used when counting money.

3   The finger joints can also become inflamed by long periods of writing. This is is most likely to be caused by gripping the pen tightly while pressing hard on the paper. Holding the pen in a relaxed fashion reduces this tension.

4   Constant over-use of the same joints, as in ballet dancing or jogging, can strain the joints in the feet.

Care of Inflamed Joints

A simple way to tell if a joint is inflamed is to feel how hot it is. It is important that you rest any inflamed joints. If you do not, then you run the risk of damaging the membrane lining the inside of the joints. In time, this damage could spread to the bones. Eventually, the joint loses its normal shape. For example, the finger joints become twisted and awkward to use. This stage of arthritis is often the result of repeated use of inflamed joints.

Don't use joints which are inflamed. Rest them as much as possible. Of course, you also need medical treatment at an early stage.

Limiting Joint Injury

Aim to reduce the stretches and strains on any troublesome joints.

1   Think hard about the way you use your joints. You could ask someone else to observe you and help you work out how the problem is made worse.

2   The next step is more difficult. If possible, modify the way you use your hands and feet at work. You may need expert advice. Special gadgets that mechanically alter the strain are sometimes available or can be devised. If you can, consider transferring to a job which is less punishing on the joints.

3   Don't carry heavy things which put a strain on the finger joints. Use a shoulder bag or a shopping trolley.

4   It is in the early stages of arthritis that you should get help in preventing the distortion of joints. There are a whole range of

appliances and gadgets which make even simple jobs easier. Specially modified cutlery, tableware, kitchen utensils, tools for d-i-y jobs, etc. are available. Jar openers and water tap turners are two examples of commonly available items. There are also gadgets for building up power in the muscles which move the joints.

The occupational therapy department at your local hospital can be contacted by your doctor for advice on such appliances.

KEY POINTS

- To minimise damage to the joints, rest them when they are inflamed. Then work out ways of using your joints so that repeated stretch doesn't produce disabling arthritis.

- Regard both the skin and joint inflammation as part and parcel of the same disturbance of the body's immunity. Therefore, take extra care of your general health.

20 *TREATMENT AND SELF-HELP*

Psoriasis has many patterns and stages of activity. Therefore, its treatment is a complex subject. Your medical advisers will need to decide on the best treatment for your particular problem. It is possible to clear the skin completely for at least a period of time.

Basic Principles

1   As a general rule, the more troublesome and persistent the rash, the more potent are the drugs used.

2   Aim not to become dependent on any particular medicine. You want the benefits and not the side-effects. Reliance on drugs can generally be reduced by protecting your

immune system and maintaining high levels of skin care. However, you should also be aware of any side-effects of the drugs prescribed for you.

Creams and Ointments

1 These are of two types. Some merely soothe the skin. Others contain one or more active drugs. A drug applied to the skin can do harm as well as good – just like drugs that are taken by mouth. Take extra care, therefore, when using drug-containing creams.

2 Be certain how frequently, and for how many days or weeks, you can keep on applying a particular cream. Always apply it according to the instructions and rub it in gently. A cotton bud can be used.

3 Allow ample time for applying the treatment. Don't rush it.

4 Among creams containing cortico-steroids, some are more potent than others. Cortico-steroid drugs can produce many side-effects. Ensure that these drugs can be used safely on the area of skin you are treating.

Apply such creams sparingly. Using large amounts doesn't speed up healing.

5 Bland ointments, such as Vaseline, can of course, be used more generously. Sometimes Vaseline stops the red patches from drying out. The best method of use is to allow about 10 minutes for the ointment to soak into the skin. You can then use tissues to wipe off any excess on the skin surface.

6 When using a product new to you, try it out on a test patch of psoriasis for a few days. Carefully read and follow the printed instructions supplied with the drug. If the psoriasis is in a highly active stage, the skin may not be able to tolerate the new drug straight away. Keep a record of any creams which might have irritated the skin.

7 It is not always necessary to use messy ointments. It may be possible to use safe and effective products that do not stain the skin or your clothes. Discuss the choice with your family doctor.

8 If there is hard skin on the surface, this must first be removed. Only then, can an active drug pass easily through to the deeper layers in the skin. Ointments containing salicylic acid are often used to remove the hard skin. Such preparations are especially important when the scalp hair has become matted. After a few days of treatment, the scales become

soft and loose and can be washed away. A lotion or a cream containing an active drug can then be applied and will penetrate the hair follicles. Remember to follow the advice on scalp care outlined in Chapter 6.

9   Don't expect the rash to disappear within a few days of starting treatment. There are no rules about how quickly the skin will respond. A period of about six to eight weeks is usual.

10 Don't lose heart if you can't treat the skin every day. However, it is important to persist with the routine until the skin is clear. The chances of psoriasis lingering on are then reduced.

Tablets or Injections

These are generally reserved for situations in which the psoriasis becomes a disability. Fortunately, this is uncommon.

The most effective of these drugs carry risks of side-effects. Aim to keep their use to the minimum. Don't ease up on general skin care and maintenance of your immune system if a drug has been used to clear your skin of psoriasis.

Patterns of Healing

1   The skin heals as a whole but some areas heal more quickly than others. Psoriasis on the arms may heal fairly quickly. Patches on the legs generally take about twice as long to respond completely. Therefore, persist with the treatment.

2   As the psoriasis heals, the white flakes on the surface disappear. The centre of the patch becomes flatter and paler. Healing then spreads outwards to the edge. In the last stage of healing, this edge can still be felt above the skin surface. Don't ease up on the treatment until the skin flattens out completely.

3   Once you notice an improvement in the rash, your self-confidence will also improve. This mental change will then itself help the healing process in the skin.

4   Even after the healing appears to be complete to the naked eye, keep up with regular treatment for a week or so. Skin changes due to inflammation deep below the skin surface also have to be reversed.

Care of Healed Skin

1   Regard treatment with creams or tablets as a method of healing the skin rapidly. Once this is achieved, treat the newly healed skin with care. It needs time to toughen up.

2   Protect healed areas from injury by friction, weather damage or irritating chemicals such as detergents. The new skin cannot retain moisture and dries out easily in cold weather. Apply a bland cream or ointment, whichever is more comfortable, as often as necessary to protect the skin.

3   If you neglect your general skin care, you could soon be back to square one. The psoriasis becomes more active again. Then, as the next step in treatment, you could be advised to use a more potent drug. Avoid this pitfall. Aim to control the condition yourself.

Alternative Remedies

Various alternative remedies have been around for decades. These include physical methods of treatment, such as acupuncture or aromatherapy, as well as herbal creams. You may want to try these out. The temptation is understandable. If possible, don't proceed without medical advice. Note, too, that someone claiming to be an expert in this field may only be exploiting your condition.

If you decide to use a herbal cream, limit the treatment to a test patch for a few days. Herbal tablets, if taken long enough, may have serious side-effects. You may need blood tests to check for these. Bear in mind, also, that what might have suited a friend or relative may not suit your skin or your particular type of psoriasis. Whenever possible, get professional advice.

KEY POINTS

- There is good and safe treatment for most types of psoriasis. Follow the instructions carefully.

- When potent drugs are recommended, take extra care of your general health as well as the skin.

- The aim of the whole exercise should be to let you get on with your life, with little or no cost to your body. Then you will have taken control of the condition.

21 *PSORIASIS: AN OVERVIEW*

This final chapter should help you think about your own skin problem from a distance. You can then plan how to adapt all the various instructions to suit yourself.

The Activity of Psoriasis: a Summary

Three factors are important in keeping psoriasis active – skin stretch, the balance of moisture in the skin, and the immune system. Key information about each of these factors is summarised here:

SKIN STRETCH

The physical source of skin stretch injury can be either inside or outside the skin.

| MOISTURE BALANCE | The skin sometimes fails to retain the moisture it needs. This causes the skin to split.
At the other extreme, some areas of the skin are in a micro-climate of warmth and humidity. Possible reasons for this are:
a) the skin is not always dried properly;
b) the fat in the body folds makes them deeper;
c) sweat builds up and the folds are not kept dry enough. |
|---|---|
| IMMUNE SYSTEM | The immune system is less effective because of mental stress or habits such as smoking. |

A Cautionary Example

Psoriasis is a far more complex problem than this book suggests. However, skin stretch, moisture balance and the immune system shape the pattern of psoriasis in most people. Together, they play the most important part in determining where on the body the rash is most troublesome and how active the psoriasis becomes.

For example, let us assume you have a stressful job, smoke 10 cigarettes a day, have low immunity and then catch a throat infection. A few days later, psoriasis appears on your body. Gradually, as the immunity recovers, most of the skin heals. However, the hair-line on the forehead becomes red and flaky as the roots get pulled. The ear-folds are also not completely dried when you shampoo your hair. The skin in the ear-folds splits and lets in bacteria, which trigger off another attack of psoriasis. Hence the importance of skin care.

Skin Care: a Summary

The range of instructions set out in this book are based on three simple rules about skin care:

1 If the inflamed skin is wet, then keep it dry. If it is dry, then moisturise it.

2 Reduce the amount of stretch on the skin to a level it can tolerate safely.

3 Try and follow a lifestyle that eases the strains on the immune system.

We don't know why otherwise normal skin responds to various injuries by producing psoriasis. However, once the rash appears, these three rules of skin care become important. While psoriasis is in its early stages, your aim is to aid the drug treatment and to check the condition from progressing. You will then have taken control of the problem for yourself.

Action Plan for Self-help

- Read again the early chapters of this book covering general skin care and immunity. Then concentrate on the various chapters that refer to the areas of your body affected by the psoriasis.

- Write down a plan of the steps you should take. List the things that you can do straight away separately from the ones that may take longer.

- Prepare yourself to be patient before you begin to notice the benefits.

- Some of the recommended modifications in your lifestyle will gradually become a matter of habit. At that stage, psoriasis will no longer be a nuisance to you.

APPENDIX 1

Self-help Groups

A lot of practical information is exchanged when these groups meet. Try and join one. There may be a group associated with your local hospital dermatology clinic.

You may also like to join a national association, which may have a local group in your area.

Psoriasis Association
7 Milton Street
Northampton, NN2 7JG
Tel: 01604 711129   Fax: 01604 792894

Psoriatic Arthropathy Alliance
136 High Street
Bushey
Herts WD2 3DJ
Tel/fax: 01923 672837

National Eczema Society
163 Eversholt Street
London NW1 1BU
Tel: 0171 388 4097   Fax: 0171 388 5882
This society produces a magazine which includes helpful advice on skin care.

APPENDIX 2

Further Reading

If you wish to read more about skin care and psoriasis, you may find the following two books interesting and useful.

Healthy Skin: The Facts
by Rona M. Mackie
Oxford University Press (1992)

This family guide gives information on skin care throughout life. It also explains fully the effect of sunlight radiation on the skin.

Coping with Psoriasis
by Ronald Marks
Sheldon Press (1994)

This book contains a discussion of the causes and the treatment of psoriasis.

APPENDIX 3

Useful Products

Your major drug treatment will of course be supervised by your doctor. Listed here are various other products you may wish to use. Before trying anything new, discuss your particular problem with the pharmacist.

SALT WASHES

A salt wash is an antiseptic as well as a method of drying the skin. Use half a teaspoonful of cooking salt to a pint of tepid water. Use cotton wool or even cotton buds to apply the salt solution to small areas of skin. For a salt bath, add about 5 tablespoonfuls of salt to the bath water. Too many salt washes make the skin dry and uncomfortable, so use them sparingly.

SUNSCREENS

Note that these provide only partial protection from the sun's rays. They also have to be regularly reapplied because they wear off due to sweating and friction. Also note that fake tans do not protect the skin at all.

Use sunscreens with an S.P.F. (Sun Protection Factor) of 15 to 25. Two effective brands are Spectraban Ultra by Steifel, and ROC 15 Total Sunblock cream (available either tinted or untinted). Sweat-proof non-greasy sunscreens are available and are good for sports such as sailing. New products appear regularly. Discuss your needs with the pharmacist.

SKIN-SHIELD

Skin-Shield by Colorsport is a coating for use on jewellery, bra hooks and watches to reduce absorption of nickel (see Chapter 18). It does wear off and has to be re-applied from time to time. Other similar products are also available.

SHAMPOOS

There are many suitable products on the market. Ceanel Concentrate by Quinoderm is effective at killing off yeasts that live in the scalp. Ask your pharmacist for advice about both medicated and mild non-medicated shampoos.

ANTI-YEAST TREATMENT

Canesten-HC Cream by Bayer is an anti-yeast treatment containing clotrimazole 1% and hydrocortisone 1%. There are also other similar products. A doctor's prescription will be needed.

The cream kills off yeasts and many of the bacteria which settle on the inflamed skin. It is useful for calming down very sore skin, especially in the body folds. If it stings, the pharmacist can dilute the cream with 50% of Aqueous Cream BP. In this form, the cream can be rubbed in the scalp and washed off very easily. It should also be rubbed under the ends of the finger-nails. The aim is to kill off the germs that thrive under the nails. Otherwise, you re-introduce them to your skin when you scratch it. Canesten Lotion is useful for inflamed nail folds.

APPENDIX 4

For Your Doctor

You may find it useful to discuss the points on these two pages with your doctor. These deal with the medical aspects of self-help care for people with psoriasis. They also clarify some of the underlying ideas in this book. The aim is to avoid confusion in the advice you receive.

THE TEXT

The advice in this book is mainly aimed at people with psoriasis which has been recently diagnosed or is at an easily manageable stage. The instructions would be less useful to the very small group of people who need long-term hospital care.

The book is essentially a collection of instruction leaflets on self-help for psoriasis. The emphasis is therefore on practical advice and not on education. Psoriasis is deliberately not referred to as a "skin disease". To the vast majority of people with psoriasis, it is a problem to be overcome and suppressed.

Many complex ideas have been set out briefly and simply. More detailed explanations might therefore help. Furthermore, it is very easy to assume that common-sense will always be used in skin care.

Some obvious facts have been deliberately emphasised. The aim throughout the book has been to establish that other people with psoriasis have also faced identical problems.

MEDICAL
MANAGEMENT

The spectrum of psoriasis is far wider than has been described here. Obviously, the advice on self-help has to be tailored to suit the individual.

Special guidance may be needed when a change of lifestyle is desired. Persisting with self-help measures can be difficult for some people. Detailed advice on coping with mental stress, alcohol and tobacco addiction may help. A knowledge of any domestic problems should make it easier to discuss together how they may influence the psoriasis. This knowledge may also help secure family support.

SUMMARY

It is not possible to offer self-help guidance that would benefit everyone with psoriasis to the same extent. Most people want to know how to reverse the chain of events which produced the rash before it becomes a major nuisance.

More often than not, psoriasis doesn't get worse without reason. The pattern of its activity is closely related to the quality of skin care and to lifestyle. It should be possible to identify the factors which make psoriasis progress to an unstable stage. (Many of these triggers are discussed in the earlier chapters on skin care.) Some people may themselves be able to work out this relationship easily. For others, professional guidance on ways of modifying skin care and lifestyle could be helpful.

INDEX

A
Action plan, for self-help, 115
Active phase, of psoriasis, 18
Acupuncture, 110-111
Alcohol, and stress, 83
Allergies, 16, 93-97
  allergic reaction, 93-94
  common, of skin, 95
  and feet, 62
  general advice, 97
  and hands, 56
  metal compounds, 95
  metal-related psoriasis, 98-100
  Skin-Shield, 119
Alternative remedies, 110-111
Anti-yeast treatment, 119
Aromatherapy, 110-111
Arthritis, 101-104

B
Baths, 34-35
Body folds
  infection and psoriasis, 21
  skin care of, 47-51
Books, further reading, 117
Brushing hair, 39, 40

C
Canesten-HC Cream, 119
Chemical fumes, 44-45

Children
  psoriasis in, 71-74
Chronic phase of psoriasis, 18
Combing hair, 39, 40
Cortico-steroids, 44, 106-107
Cosmetics, 35
  skin allergies, 35, 95
Creams, 106-108
  Canesten-HC, 119
  herbal, 111
Cuticles, care of, 53

D
Deodorants, 35
Dermatitis, 56
Detergents, and hands, 56
Diet, 89-92
  and nickel allergy, 100
  skin responses to food, 96
Doctor, discussing self-help
  with your, 120-121
Dormant phase of psoriasis, 18
Drugs
  skin responses, 96
  and sun-sensitivity, 67
Drying the skin, 34, 57

E
Ear-folds, 39
Ear-piercing, and metal
  allergy, 99

Ears, skin care of, 40-41
Eczema Society, National, 116
Exercise, and psoriasis, 91
Exercises, for legs, 37
Eyebrows, 44
Eyelashes, 44

F
Face, 43-46
  general care of, 43-45
  shaving, 43
  weather protection, 45
Family matters, 75-78
Family support, 76-77
Feet, skin care of, 59-64
Female hormones, and
  psoriasis, 77-78
Food
  skin responses, 96
  see also Diet
Footwear, 61-62
  for children, 72

G
Gadgets, and limiting joint
  injury, 103-104
Gloves, and hand care, 57
Groin, skin care of, 49-50

H
Hair, matted, 41
Hair care, 40-41
Hair removal, 35
Hair-line, 39

Hands, skin care of, 52-58
Healing, patterns of, 109
Herbal creams, 111
Holidays, 69
Hormones, female, and
  psoriasis, 77-78
Hormone replacement therapy
  (HRT), 78
Housewife's eczema, 56
Humidity, 21, 33, 44
Hypoallergenic products, 35

I
Immunity, 28-31
  in children, 73
  immune responses in
    psoriasis, 29
  immune system and the skin, 28
  influences on, 30-31
  and lifestyle, 30
  and relaxation, 87
  and skin healing, 29-30
  and smoking, 85-88
Inheritance and psoriasis, 75
Injections, 108
Itching, control of, 33

J
Jewellery, and psoriasis, 16,
  99-100
Joints
  care of, 101-104
  limiting injury, 103-104
  patterns of strain, 101-102

and the skin, 86
Soap, 34
Soles of feet, care of, 59-61
Split skin, 48-49
Standing, and psoriasis, 36
Stress, 79-84
  and alcohol, 83
  chemical mechanism, 80
  and family support, 76-77
  general advice, 82
  and the menopause, 78
  and psoriasis in children, 73
  and sleep, 82
  and smoking, 87
Stretched skin, and psoriasis,
 20, 112
Sun-sensitivity, 66-67
Sunbed, 66
Sunburn, and psoriasis, 67
Sunlight, 65-70
  effect on face, 45
  and holidays, 69
  influence on psoriasis, 65
  protection from, 68-69
  and skin healing, 66
Sunscreens, 68-69, 118-119
Support, from family, 76-77
Support bandages, 37
Swimming, 35, 72

T
Teenagers, 76
Throat infection, and
 psoriasis, 21, 86

Toe nails, 62-63
Toe-webs, 62-63
Treatments, 105-111
  alternative remedies, 110-111
  basic principles, 105-106
  creams and ointments, 106-108
  patterns of healing, 109
  and self-help, 15
  tablets or injections, 108

U
Underwear, 49
Unstable phase of psoriasis, 18

V
Vaginal discharge, 50
Varicose veins, 36
Vaseline, 107
  use before swimming, 35
Vegetarians, 91

W
Watch strap, 99
Weather protection, 36
Weight, and psoriasis, 89-90
Wet-wiping, 50
Wind, effect on face, 45

Y
Yeasts, 16
  anti-yeast treatment, 119

Z
Zinc, 83, 91

PRIORITY ORDER FORM

Cut out or photocopy this form and send it (post free in the UK) to:

Class Publishing Customer Service
FREEPOST (no stamp needed)
LONDON W6 7BR

Tel: 01752 202 301

Fax: 01752 202 333

Please send me urgently
(tick boxes below)

**Post included
price per copy
(UK only)**

☐ **Skin care for psoriasis**
(ISBN 1 872362 63 X) £10.95

☐ **Your child's epilepsy: a parents' guide**
(ISBN: 1 872362 61 3) £12.95

☐ **Asthma at your fingertips**
(ISBN: 1 872362 06 0) £14.95

☐ **Allergies at your fingertips**
(ISBN: 1 872362 52 4) £14.95

☐ **High blood pressure at your fingertips**
(ISBN 1 872362 48 6) £14.95

☐ **Diabetes at your fingertips**
(ISBN: 1 872362 49 4) £14.95

☐ **Cancer information at your fingertips**
(ISBN: 1 872362 56 7) £14.95

TOTAL: _____

Easy ways to pay
Cheque: I enclose a cheque payable to Class Publishing for £_____
Credit card: please debit my ☐ Access ☐ Visa ☐ Amex ☐ Switch

Number: _____ Expiry date: _____

Name: _____

Address: _____

Town: _____ County: _____ Postcode: _____

My telephone number (in case of queries): _____

Class Publishing's guarantee: remember that if, for any reason, you are not satisfied with these books, we will refund all your money, without any questions asked. Prices and VAT rates may be altered for reasons beyond our control.

Ref: SCFP97